My First Investment in Health for Kids and Teens

What is sleep, exercise, diet and why do I need it?

from various sources. Please consult a licensed professional before attempting any techniques outlined in this book.

By reading this document, the reader agrees that under no circumstances is the author responsible for any losses, direct or indirect, that are incurred as a result of the use of the information contained within this document, including, but not limited to, errors, omissions, or inaccuracies.

Table of Contents

Introduction: Formative Years

There are many books on the market that indicate how a parent can deal with their child through that child's teenage years, but the people who should really be learning about what to expect during these formative years are those actually undergoing them—in other words, you.

As a parent, and someone who has worked with hundreds of children in their formative years, I have heard many arguments that play into the moody teenager scenario. What I have realized after working with kids of all ages is that tweens and teens are given a really bad reputation; one that they do not deserve.

Of all the age groups, those between the ages of 11 to 18 years go through more changes in a short period of time than any other age group. In a matter of eight to ten years, generally speaking, teenagers go from being a child to an adult; from having almost everything done for them, to being responsible for taking care of themselves, and navigating their future.

As a teenager, your body is going through physical, mental, and emotional changes that are not only exhausting, but a bit scary to go through as well. There are changes in your cognition, body, and perspective, and the best way to navigate through these uncharted times is to become an advocate for yourself, and understand what you will be going through, so that you can invest in your health.

Emotional and physical health are directly related, and if one is not nourished, the other will likely falter. Caring for emotional, physical, and mental health independently will help in all these facets but understanding how to foster all of your body's needs from the inside out is how you will maintain a healthy lifestyle, even into adulthood.

There are several aspects that come together to form a healthy mind, strong body, and emotional wellbeing. Our habits, our personal connections, and the way we see our worth all contribute to how we see and feel about ourselves and others. Understanding what you need to do to be healthy and learning how your changing body and mind will affect aspects of those needs, will ultimately help you make informed decisions.

What is healthy?

It would be nice if there was an exact formula for being healthy, but everyone is different, so we just have to navigate through ups and downs, until we find out what works well for each of us individually. According to the World Health Organization (WHO), physical and mental health contribute to overall wellness.

You may have heard the term "body mass index," or BMI, in gym class. This measure helps determine whether or not you are overweight, but this does not actually give us an accurate account of one's overall health. Health consists of many aspects that come together to make up your wellness.

How psychological and physical health are related

Physical and mental health affect each other in cycles and are connected by chemistry of the body. Your mood is affected by things that occur around you, but the emotions are created from neurotransmitters in the brain, as well as from hormones. The brain is sent chemicals through these transmitters that tell you to feel sad, happy, or worried. When the neurotransmitters are not firing properly because of a lack of serotonin or dopamine, this can lead to anxiety or depression.

Mental health affects the body

When a person suffers from mental illness, this can affect the health of the body, since it becomes stressed, and can lead to heart disease and other illnesses brought on by worry, such as ulcers.

By taking care of our mental health, we can improve our body's physical health by eating nutritious meals, exercising, and getting a good night's sleep. The brain is able to rebalance the chemicals and help restore a more stable mindset.

During the teenage years, there are challenges and changes that make it difficult to always keep a positive mindset, and to maintain an adequate level of physical activity. To balance the mind and body, and have them create a healthier outlook together, you need to understand what is changing in your body, what the cognitive and physical changes and needs of your body are, and how nutrition plays an important role in all of this.

Cognitive growth

By the age of 15, you will have the same abilities to think logically as an adult. These abilities are developed significantly from the age of around seven, when a child is first capable of determining what will happen in a given situation and can anticipate a possible outcome. This matures significantly between the ages of 12 to 15, but it is remarkable that it begins at such a young age. These rational thinking skills develop in the following areas:

1. Memory

The ability to remember spontaneously learned information, as well as the ability to remember long-term.

2. Attention

The ability to focus on one stimulant improves, even when there are other distractions present. The ability to successfully pay attention to more than one thing at a time improves, too, and multi-tasking skills develop.

3. Organization

This is when kids are able to use mnemonic devices to become more organized and to strategize more efficiently.

4. Processing

The speed at which you think rapidly improves between the ages of 5 and 15, and then begins to level off.

5. Metacognition

This is the awareness of thought processes, and the recognition of understanding that goes into them. Although there is a lot of cognitive development that goes on in these early years, the brain is not thought to be fully developed until the age of 21 to 23.

Hypothetical thinking

One of the greatest developments in adolescence is deductive reasoning skills which lead to hypothetical thinking. While children think in black and white, based on what they see and know, an adolescent can think of the possibilities of what may happen, and give them the ability to make plans in the future, foresee consequences, and be able to determine various reasons for events.

Teenagers can convey their point of view with well-thought-out examples, because they have the ability to see beyond what is obviously there. The brain in adolescence is able to consider possibilities beyond what is immediately present and come up with alternate realities and scenarios.

Realistic thinking

As children, we are able to accept the most fantastical scenarios and are ready to believe most things that we hear. In adolescent years, we question situations and stories that we do not consider to be realistic. The ability to determine what is real and what is not, comes with maturity and brain development that is sharpened in the teenage years.

This part of maturity will differentiate between fantasy and real-life, although entertaining a good urban legend now and then isn't going to affect your ability to perform realistic thinking.

Metacognition

Metacognition is when an adolescent becomes aware of their thought process and how it works. This regulatory system allows you to control how you think, and helps you understand the learning process behind it.

Becoming wiser

The ability to use judgment based on experiences is developed primarily between the ages of 14-25. When people refer to a wise old man, they may be right in the sense that the old man is wise, but he would have gained most of his wisdom in the earlier years of his life. Our learning potential is virtually limitless, so people learn throughout their whole lives, but wisdom and intelligence are two very different things.

Psychological development

Psychological development refers to the cognitive, intellectual, social, and emotional capacity of people throughout the span of their lives.

Identify formation

The formation of one's identity, or identity development, is one of the most important stages of development in an adolescent. This is how you see yourself and determine the type of person you are, and who you want to become.

Identity

Identity is everything to an individual because it is the feeling of who we are. Identities are developed based on our experiences in life, who we spend time with, and what our environment provides for us. If you live in a mansion in Beverly Hills, your environment will help to mold your identity, just as living in a small village will form your sense of self in a completely different way. Your identity can change over time, depending on your changing social and economical state.

Our self-identity is how we see ourselves. Our perception of ourselves can change depending on our social groups and how we perceive our family, friends, school, and how we feel we belong. Our self-identity is greatly based on how we perceive ourselves and our own worth.

Social identity is how others see us, and can be based on many factors, such as:

- ethnicity and race
- gender
- social status
- sexual orientation

Sexual identity

Sexual identity can be a large determining factor in how comfortable we are with ourselves, or in our surroundings. Adolescence is a time when many realize their sexual identity, and whether they are cisgender, bisexual, transgender, non-binary, or otherwise.

There are several factors that play into the emotional and mental perceptions, as well as the wellness of an adolescent. The first step in the investment of your health is to understand what you are going through during these formative years, and how you can help keep your body and mind in optimal health.

We will go through various ways to support your brain, body, and emotional development, and help you to maintain optimal health throughout these formative years. Your first step was to show interest in your personal health, and you should be commended for that. You, the youth, are our most important piece to the future, and you deserve to be educated about your health, and be informed about all that you will be going through in the coming years.

Chapter 1: Needs Change as You Grow

Everyone has needs that change over time as they develop, learn, and grow to become different people. Tweens and teenagers change at such a rapid rate that you are constantly evolving into a more wise and independent version of yourself. As you continue to change, your needs as an individual will grow with you.

As homosapiens, we all have needs for basic survival, including water and food, but there is also the need for belonging, independence, and fun, which applies to youth more than anyone. During adolescence, there is tremendous emotional growth, and a need to be accepted socially. All tweens and teens want to feel like they belong among their peers and are included in social activities and social interactions. The tween and teen years are a time when a child wants to be seen as more of an equal in the eyes of their parents, teachers, and other adult figures in their life.

As a teenager, you may feel the need to belong more, as the years go on. Seeing friends spur off into different groups, fueling varying interests from yours, or becoming more social than you, can be intimidating and stressful. As your needs change, so will you. It is important that you make decisions based on what is best for you, and not for others.

Belonging

As a teen gets older, their freedom grows, and the opportunity to do different things with their friends changes. Instead of going to a friend's house to watch a movie or play a video game, you may be invited to a party, or to go bowling, both of which can be perfectly safe. As your social network grows and changes, you will be forced to make some big decisions.

Your friends may get into drugs, vandalism, or may skip school because they can't be bothered. Your decision might be whether to go along with your friends in order to fit in, or to step away from that social connection, so you can make better choices.

Decisions

It can be frustrating when a teenager isn't given the option to make choices that involve their own life, such as where they live, what they eat, or how free time is spent. If you are being controlled in your life, and not able to make your own decisions, it might be time to talk to your parents or guardians about giving you more control.

Everyone needs to be responsible for decisions so they can learn and grow, including you. Ask to help with buying groceries or making dinner, or offering input into where you go on vacation, in order to feel like you have some control over your life. When you're older, you can run your own life, and will in fact be expected to, so it will help you to make some decisions now, before that time comes, or you may be clueless as to what to expect.

Independence

There are rules that many teenagers must abide by in their homes, such as completing chores, following a curfew, being respectful, and participating in family activities. There is also an urge and need to become more independent by going out on your own with friends, making decisions that affect your future, or even being trusted to take the car out once you get your license.

Independence is a big part of becoming an adult, but to earn that right, you need to be held accountable to your word. If you ask to go to a party and say you won't drink, then you actually need to refrain from drinking. If you ask to take the car out and promise not to drive unsafely, then you should do just that, and not get a speeding ticket or other driving infraction.

In order to gain independence, proving you are as good as your word will get you a long way. You can gain the trust of your parents and other authority figures by being true to your promises.

Pre-Pubescent Years

The words "pre-pubescent" and "puberty" usually bring on a few belly laughs, but it is a complicated time that brings on more changes than you will ever go through in such a short period of time, in any other part of your life. There are different stages to puberty, and it helps to know what they all are, so you can understand what is happening to your changing body.

Everyone goes through puberty at different times, and there is no right or wrong time, nor is there a stage you should be at, at a given age. Everyone develops at a different rate, simply when their body is ready. The average age when a child begins to go through puberty is 11 for girls, and 12 for boys, and it takes about four years to be complete. However, it's worth knowing that children have been known to begin puberty as early as 8 years old, and as late as 14 years old.

Talking about puberty can be awkward for some parents, but it is nothing to be ashamed of. So that you can understand what you are going through, I have outlined the path of puberty that most girls and boys go through on their journey to becoming adults. The stages and development vary for everyone, and your experience may not be the same as everyone else's. If you are concerned about any part of your pre-pubescent or puberty growth, talk to your parents, or to a doctor.

Some of the signs to recognize as the beginning of puberty include:

For girls: early signs of puberty

The first indication that a girl is entering puberty is that she will begin to develop breasts. It is common for there to be discomfort and tenderness in the chest area, and one breast may be more developed than the other, but each will even out over time.

You will also notice pubic hair beginning to grow, and there may be an increase in hair on your arms and legs.

Midway signs of puberty

After one year, and for a duration of one to two years, a girl may notice the following changes occurring with her in body:

- first period (about two years after puberty begins)
- breasts continue to develop, and become fuller
- pubic hair becomes curlier and more coarse
- hair begins to grow in other parts of the body, such as the armpits, and some girls may find they have hair on their upper lip (this is normal)
- you may find that you sweat more
- vaginal discharge that is white (also completely normal)
- acne may develop in the form of black/white heads, or puss-filled pockets
- weight gain is common, and you will likely find that you have more fat than usual, and begin to

fill out in your hips (this weight gain is normal, and necessary for proper growth)

- a growth spurt usually occurs of about two to three inches, between the beginning of your first period, and over the next couple of years, when you will reach the height that you will be as an adult

While many of these changes may seem unpleasant, it is all a natural part of your body developing and growing, so that you can become a healthy adult. This can be a difficult time when you are more developed than others, or if you haven't begun developing by a certain age. Remember to stay positive, and know that at some point all women go through this stage, and it is nothing to be ashamed of.

The weight gain that you may see in yourself is also completely normal, and is a result of your hormones igniting changes in your physical appearance. This is not the time to diet or feel inadequate; you need the extra weight to distribute to the various parts of your body that are changing, developing, and growing.

Later signs of puberty

In the last stages of puberty, the girl will be very much as she will be in adulthood. Breasts are developed, pubic hair is filled in and can grow along the top of the inner thighs, and the genitals are developed. You also will likely not grow any taller.

For boys: early signs of puberty

As with girls, there are different ages that boys will reach puberty. Early signs of puberty in boys is that the skin around the scrotum becomes thinner and more red, and the testicles and penis will become larger. Pubic hair will begin to grow around the base of the penis.

Midway signs of puberty

After about one year, and for the following one to two years, the changes in a boy might include:

- scrotum becomes darker
- testicles and penis will grow
- pubic hair becomes curlier and more coarse
- hair begins to grow under armpits
- may notice swollen breasts
- you may find that you sweat more
- voice may crack as a result of the voice changing to become deeper
- may experience involuntary ejaculation during sleep (this is normal)
- may develop acne in the form of white/blackheads, or puss-filled pockets
- will grow in height by around three inches per year
- muscles begin to develop

Late signs of puberty

In the last stages of puberty, a male's genitals will develop to the size they will be as an adult, and pubic hair will continue to grow, and may spread to the upper, inner thighs. Facial hair will grow darker, and he will need to consider whether to shave or not. His height potential will be nearly complete by the time he reaches 16 years of age, but he may continue very slow growth until around age 18.

The changes both males and females see and feel may be awkward at times, but remember it is completely natural, and that you are not the only one who has gone through, or will be going through these changes. Understanding the different stages of puberty will help you to be more prepared for these changes, and understand what is happening to your body.

Growth spurt

Most kids have heard of a growth spurt, which indicates a large change in the size or height of someone or something, in a very short period of time. To put it in simple terms, puberty is really about having a growth spurt, only it's every aspect of yourself, including the body, brain, and emotions, as each rapidly grows and changes.

During puberty, the growth that you go through can be significant in a short period of time, which often results in clumsiness, since you are not used to the length of your rapidly growing arms, feet, and height.

As mentioned above, your body changes as the hips become fuller for girls, and boys become more muscular, and many other changes occur. With extra curves, and significant changes in your body and vocal changes, there's no one that is safe from feeling insecure from time to time.

Acne

Acne is common in teenagers, because the changing hormones make the skin more oily. Acne may be troubling, and can pop up on your face, back, and arms, and it can be itchy, sore, and make the skin appear blotchy. According to dermatologists, the best way to care for your skin is to use warm (not hot) water, and a mild soap, or none at all If you suffer from severe acne and it is affecting the way you interact with others and how you feel about yourself, it may be worth it to talk to your doctor about a possible solution.

Body odor

It is hard to consider puberty as a beautiful time when your body is going through so many awkward changes that make you feel different, and often less than beautiful. Another very natural and common part of going through puberty is that you may develop body odor, especially under your armpits. The glands found in your skin are activated by the hormones that are released during puberty, including sweat glands, which account for the funky odor from your skin when you sweat.

The best way to help control the odor is to shower daily, and make sure you put on clean clothes every day, as well as use deodorant to help prevent the smell that comes with sweating. Remember that this is a common issue for many teenagers, and that in time, it should subside.

Recognizing yourself

One of the biggest challenges that come along with puberty is that you may seem as different on the inside as you do on the outside. The mood swings that are caused by hormones are likely to direct your personality at times before you are able to stop them, or even understand what is going on. You may feel scared and strange, and it only becomes more frustrating when others think that you are being irrational or moody.

The changes you are experiencing are new to you and everyone around you. Your temper, patience, and personality are all contouring, growing, and melding together, to help bring you to a place that you will feel comfortable in your new body and mind.

Sex talk

Part of taking care of your emotional and physical self is to understand everything that is going on with your entire body and mind during this exciting and tumultuous time. One of the biggest changes you will notice is that you will likely begin to have sexual feelings, which can be confusing. You may have already become sexually physical, or have thought about it, which is natural.

The best thing you can do for your health is to understand what is going on at this stage in development. Talking to your parents about sex, or finding another trusted adult is going to benefit you, and keep you from making decisions that you may regret later on.

Protecting yourself emotionally from a partner, and also from sexually transmitted diseases, is crucial. You may consider yourself too mature to need advice about sex, but if you want to be in control of your overall health, you need to have the difficult talk with someone in your life, such as a parent or doctor.

The Teenage Years

It is very important to me that teenagers have their own guide to who they are becoming, the changes they are going through, and how to deal with their ever-changing selves.

Many of the developments you undergo as a teenager affect how you think and feel about yourself and toward others. Essentially, the changes that you experience can make you feel that you are inadequate, that you don't belong, or that you are not enough. As the mother of three teenagers, I can tell you that you are amazing, and everything you are going through is extremely difficult emotionally, physically, and mentally.

Many adults forget what it is like to be judged by your peers, or to try your best, only to be told it wasn't good enough. Because you are still considered a child by many, you are not treated with the respect you deserve, despite the massive changes you have undergone, and the strides you have taken toward becoming an active member of society.

Teenagers have many questions because they, and the people around them, are constantly changing. It's easy to forget the trauma that adolescence goes through during the journey toward adulthood. When you don't understand your feelings, or the reactions of those around you, consider the following:

Your change affects others

It is not uncommon for people to feel offended when someone changes, and this includes your parents. You are becoming more independent and making your own decisions, which can be difficult for any parent to accept.

While unfair at times, consider this: Your parents raised you from birth, when you knew how to breathe and cry on your own, but little else. They have spent more than a decade taking care of you, providing for you, making your decisions, and keeping you safe, and now you are branching out on your own, and little by little, they are losing control.

Losing control of a child does not affect most parents, because they want to keep their child under their thumb, but rather, it scares them because they are unable to make sure that their child is protected and safe in the big world that they know so well to be unfair. If your parents are limiting your time away from them, or preventing you from making your own decisions, you might need to sit them down, and remind them of all the good decisions you have made, and that you are changing and growing because of the good job they have done as parents.

Communication is often the key to moving beyond restrictions and misunderstandings. While discussing your potential for less limitations in your life, make your point, but also listen to the concerns of your parents, because they love you, and are concerned for your safety.

You do deserve the chance to make your own decisions and should be allowed more responsibilities if you have proven yourself to be a good student, you help out at home, follow rules, and genuinely try to make the right decisions. Remembering that it may be difficult for your parents to let go will help you understand that it may not be that they don't trust you, but rather, that they don't trust those around you in the world.

You are not alone

Imagine hundreds, if not thousands, of kids going through what you are right now; it's all true. If you are in junior high or high school, there is likely not one student around you that is not confused by feelings, stunned by their growth, and dealing with peer pressures and changes in social groups.

When you feel confused about why a friend may have taken something the wrong way, consider how you may have felt lately, for what others called no good reason.

As is discussed later on in this book, with the hormone changes in a teenager, as well as a mind that is still developing and maturing, it is easy to misinterpret someone's benign comment toward you as a snide remark, or a criticism.

Before you jump to conclusions, ask your friend, or whomever you believe was disrespectful, to sit down, and discuss any possible misinterpretation. More times than not, you will realize that no disrespect was meant, and that you are all just going through a really difficult and emotional time together.

It will get easier

Feeling confused, angry, anxious, sad, and an array of other difficult emotions is normal when you are going through puberty. Feeling out of control will likely not always be the case, and it may be easier for you to remind yourself that there are others who are floundering as well.

We can often misidentify depression as anger or hostility when it is really sadness and frustration that is fueling your emotions. If you feel that you are angry most of the time, then it may be a sign that you are depressed.

If you feel like life is too difficult to carry on, you need to speak to someone about those feelings. It is common to feel down for a short period of time, but if you find that there is no reprieve in your despair, speak to an adult, since it may be beneficial to get some professional help.

Chapter 2: The Layers of Sleep

Sleep is of critical importance for several reasons. Sleep is our body's time to rejuvenate, so that it can get us through the next day. At night, our body analyzes the thoughts and sights that have surrounded us through the day, from what we ate, to glimpses caught in the corner of our eyes. Sleep is when our body mends cells and recharges, much like a rechargeable battery, a cell phone, or a wireless remote.

To function at full capacity, we need to get an ample amount of sleep; but not all sleep is created equal. There are layers of sleep in which your body is at varying stages of consciousness, and both are very necessary for each of us to fall into during each sleep cycle.

It may seem hard to believe, but your body and mind are busy for the entire time you are sleeping by:

- filtering and storing information
- your nervous system making sure all systems are communicating well
- your body restoring damaged cells and re-energizing

Our bodies are amazing, so it pays off to treat them like the machines they are, by giving yourself a good eight to ten hours of sleep per night and allowing yourself to fall into the five—yes, five—different sleep cycles. There are two main stages of sleep that are most important: rapid eye movement (REM), and non-rapid eye movement stages. You may have seen someone in REM sleep, or even a pet, when their eyes dart around beneath the eyelids, and they look like they're having a wild dream, which they likely are, as this is the stage where dreams happen.

What are the five stages of sleep that you are blissfully unaware of? Let's explore what they are, and how they aid in the replenishment of your body's cells, energy, and well-being.

Stage 1

The first stage of sleep is the light stage, wherein your body and mind gently shut down, and your body feels relaxed and drowsy. This first stage of sleep typically lasts about ten minutes and is when you are most likely to be awoken by small noises or lights in the hallway.

Stage 2

Stage 2 is still a light sleep, but the body relaxes further, the muscles relax, and brain activity decreases, as it prepares for a well-deserved slumber. The second stage of sleep is where it is thought that sensory processing and memory storage occurs. In studies, brain waves spike during this time (also referred to as sleep spindles), so it has been deduced that this may be the time in which our memories are created.

Stage 3 and 4

In stages 3 and 4 of the sleep cycle, people fall into a progressively deeper sleep, and are often difficult to wake up. Your heart rate and breathing decrease in this stage of sleep, and you are completely relaxed, with your muscles limp. If you've heard the expression from your parents that you "sleep like the dead," then this would be the cycle that you are in at that time when they tried to wake you.

This is the stage of sleep that is important for your body to mend itself when it is sick, or if you have suffered an injury. During this stage, your immune system kicks into high gear, and your muscles and tissues begin to repair themselves more efficiently than they could during your awake hours.

Stage 5

Stage 5 of sleep is known as the REM stage and is by far the most entertaining stage of sleep. REM stage is most likely the stage that you will dream, your eyes dart around as mentioned, your heart can beat quickly and irregularly, and your muscles become essentially paralyzed. If you have ever had a dream that you were being chased but couldn't run, it's likely because you were in the REM phase of sleep, and your muscles literally couldn't move, so you were stuck in your dream.

Aside from the sporadic jolts and jerks that your body does during this final stage, it is also an important time for the brain, because this is where your long-term memories are formed. This is the time that the brain interprets and stores information, making it available for you to access at a later time.

Why Sleep Is Important to Our Development

Sleep is essential to everyone's development, especially teenagers, as these later years bridging adolescence and adulthood are exceptionally formative. A teenager will undergo changes in the body and brain that will translate to their adult years, help form their personality, help them to perform well in school, and regulate their emotions. Sleep helps teenagers perform optimally in all ways, but they are less likely to get the proper amount of sleep than any other age group.

As a teenager, you need between eight to ten hours of sleep every night, according to the National Sleep Foundation, in order to help with physical health, as well as emotional stability and academic achievements. How sleep affects these areas of a teen's life may seem insignificant, but they are critical, especially in the following areas:

Academics

When you get a good night's sleep, your brain is able to pay attention for greater spans of time, memory is sharper, and analytical thinking is not challenged. When you get enough sleep, you are likely to make better decisions, and you will think more creatively. Thoughts may appear crisper and come to you more easily. Decisions will also seem less difficult to make, and you will be able to retain information you may need for a test.

Emotional well-being

It can be very apparent when someone doesn't have a good night's sleep, both in attention span and focus, and in their attitude in general. Someone that doesn't sleep well can act cranky and have a difficult time accepting even the slightest obstacles throughout their day. Being on edge can cause you to overreact to a social or family situation, and make you feel that things are horribly wrong with a friend, or your parents, when others will be unaware there is a situation at all.

Prolonged periods of little or interrupted sleep can lead to depression, anxiety, and dark thoughts. The mental anguish that comes with sleep deprivation can lead to mental health problems, and cause severe rifts in personal relationships, and how you feel about yourself.

Careless behavior

The frontal lobe in the brain is responsible for decision-making. When a developing brain is deprived of sleep, it can lead to a lack of impulse control. Teenagers who are sleep deprived are more likely to make careless decisions, such as failing to wear a helmet while skateboarding or riding a bike, trying drugs or alcohol, or picking fights with others.

The frontal lobe is where our spontaneity, judgment, impulse control, and our emotional judgements are formed. Without proper sleep, the development of this critical part of the brain may lead to bad decisions that can get you into trouble.

Physical well-being

Sleep is especially important if you are physically active. Sleep aids tissue recovery and mending muscles, as well as regulating hormones, and helping to build up immune systems so you recover much quicker from injuries or ailments. Research conducted at the National Library of Medicine has determined that youth who lack sufficient sleep may be at risk for diabetes or cardiovascular conditions when they are older.

Preventing injuries

Sleep has been associated with injuries and even death in teenagers, when it comes to driving while drowsy. When you are groggy, you do not make the best decisions, and this can be when you drive, ride a bike, play sports, or anything physical that comes with risk of injury. When you are not operating with a clear and rested mind, you are endangering yourself and others.

sharper, and analytical thinking is not challenged. When you get enough sleep, you are likely to make better decisions, and you will think more creatively. Thoughts may appear crisper and come to you more easily. Decisions will also seem less difficult to make, and you will be able to retain information you may need for a test.

Emotional well-being

It can be very apparent when someone doesn't have a good night's sleep, both in attention span and focus, and in their attitude in general. Someone that doesn't sleep well can act cranky and have a difficult time accepting even the slightest obstacles throughout their day. Being on edge can cause you to overreact to a social or family situation, and make you feel that things are horribly wrong with a friend, or your parents, when others will be unaware there is a situation at all.

Prolonged periods of little or interrupted sleep can lead to depression, anxiety, and dark thoughts. The mental anguish that comes with sleep deprivation can lead to mental health problems, and cause severe rifts in personal relationships, and how you feel about yourself.

Careless behavior

The frontal lobe in the brain is responsible for decision-making. When a developing brain is deprived of sleep, it can lead to a lack of impulse control. Teenagers who are sleep deprived are more likely to make careless decisions, such as failing to wear a helmet while skateboarding or riding a bike, trying drugs or alcohol, or picking fights with others.

The frontal lobe is where our spontaneity, judgment, impulse control, and our emotional judgements are formed. Without proper sleep, the development of this critical part of the brain may lead to bad decisions that can get you into trouble.

Physical well-being

Sleep is especially important if you are physically active. Sleep aids tissue recovery and mending muscles, as well as regulating hormones, and helping to build up immune systems so you recover much quicker from injuries or ailments. Research conducted at the National Library of Medicine has determined that youth who lack sufficient sleep may be at risk for diabetes or cardiovascular conditions when they are older.

Preventing injuries

Sleep has been associated with injuries and even death in teenagers, when it comes to driving while drowsy. When you are groggy, you do not make the best decisions, and this can be when you drive, ride a bike, play sports, or anything physical that comes with risk of injury. When you are not operating with a clear and rested mind, you are endangering yourself and others.

Sleep disorders

Less common, but a possible reason for sleep disruption could be sleep disorders such as restless leg syndrome, which make your legs feel like they are being pricked, tickled, pulled, or itched from the inside, and can make it difficult to get to sleep or stay asleep.

Electronics

Since most electronics such as cell phones, video games, and laptops are used by kids and teens for stimulation, it makes it difficult for the mind to calm down to a state of lucidity so that you can relax and get a good night's sleep. Your mind will likely be wired, and firing off various situations that it experienced while online, making it difficult to fall asleep.

You know why sleep is so important, but that doesn't help you if you have difficulty falling asleep and staying asleep long enough to fulfill all of the sleep cycles. Fortunately, there are some ways that you can improve your chances of getting a better night's sleep.

1. Routine

Sticking to a routine for bedtime and waking up is going to help your body regulate and respond to a sleep schedule. Go to bed and wake up at the same time every day, including on weekends, so that your body will acclimate to a time when it becomes ready to sleep, and also prepare to become awake and alert in the morning.

2. Power Down

Whether you realize it or not, electronics such as television, cell phones, video games, or laptops will over-stimulate your mind, and make it more difficult to fall asleep. About an hour before you are going to bed, try reading for a bit, or taking a relaxing bath to help settle your mind.

3. Avoid Sugary or Caffeinated Drinks

Before bedtime, you want to avoid any drinks that have caffeine in them, or are high in sugar, as these will both keep you awake. To be safe, stick to water or decaffeinated tea, or you will be in for a sleepless night.

4. Avoid Exercise

Physical activity is a necessity to a healthy life, but not right before bed. Exercising during the day will help you sleep better, but if you exercise too close to bedtime, you will be overstimulated and unable to fall asleep.

5. A Bed Is for Sleep

A garage is to keep a car, a kitchen is where food is stored, and a bed is where you sleep, so avoid using your resting place for any other activities other than sleeping. Set up a desk for homework or playing video games, rather than sitting in your bed. If you only sleep in your bed, then your mind will automatically relax when you tuck yourself in.

Chapter 3: Why Diet Matters

Have you ever heard the expression "you are what you eat"? You are not going to walk around looking like a salad or a piece of fish, but your body—inside and out—will be reflective of the foods you consume. Every kid and teenager should learn how to take accountability for their own health early on, so that those healthy habits are set as a way of life. As a kid, you are expected to be accountable for many things, including getting up for school, doing chores and homework, and making responsible decisions, so why shouldn't you be able to hold yourself and those in your home accountable for good eating habits?

When your body and mind is still developing, it is important that you eat the right foods to help your bones, organs, and mind grow to their full potential. As a growing being, you are literally feeding your potential when you eat foods, so make sure your choices aren't limited to junk foods. Below are some of the reasons that eating a healthy diet is so important:

1. Clearer complexion

Eating healthy foods will help your skin become and stay clearer. A diet that is high in processed sugars and unhealthy fats is going to give you more break-outs than a diet that is rich in complex carbs and lean protein. Eating fruits, vegetables, fish, and other healthy foods will give you a glowing complexion; just

Deadlines and commitments

As a teenager, or even as someone approaching their teenage years, you know that pressures mount when school assignments are due, tests are upcoming, and social commitments bog down your time.

When you have an exam to study for and homework due, you may feel that you don't have enough time on an average day, and therefore you stay up later to finish what is a pressing issue. This eats into your sleep schedule and makes it difficult to get a full night's rest. In addition to not having enough time in the 14-16 hour day, you may feel overwhelmed and stressed with deadlines and social commitments to friends, which can make it increasingly difficult to fall asleep.

Anxiety and depression

If you suffer from anxiety or depression, you may already have difficulty sleeping, because your mind is constantly feeding you with thoughts that are depleting your mental health, which in turn adds to sleep issues, and can lead to insomnia.

ADHD and other neurodivergent disorders

Attention deficit hyperactivity disorder (ADHD), autism, and Tourette' syndrome are only a few neurodivergent disorders that can cause sleep disruptions in adolescence. Not only can these conditions lend to difficulty sleeping, but sleep can also make these disorders more pronounced.

How to Sleep Better

Sleep is essential for the proper development of a child or teenager, but the National Center for Biotechnology Information suggests that the majority of adolescents are getting fewer than eight hours per night. The lack of sleep is more prevalent in males than females and is considerably higher in teens than any other age group.

There is not one reason associated with teenagers lacking sufficient sleep, but there are some factors that could play an important part, which is also accountable for a lack of sleep in adolescence.

Staggered wake and sleep schedules

The circadian rhythm is the 24 hour cycle that a body goes through in a day, including wake and sleep times, and everything in between. A teenager tends to have the impulse to sleep later at night when their bodies release melatonin, a natural chemical that the body produces and releases when it is time to go to sleep.

Since melatonin is released later in teens, their cycle can become hindered when they have to wake up early the next morning for school, leaving them feeling tired. This cycle will repeat itself until the weekend, when many teens try to catch up on their sleep, only to make it more difficult to fall asleep at a decent hour, and wake up bright and early on Monday morning.

steer clear of pop, chips, doughnuts, and other unhealthy foods.

2. Energy

Eating healthy foods will give you more energy for playing sports or participating in extracurricular activities. Our bodies run on the calories we consume by turning them into energy, and the types of foods matter. If we only eat sugary, carb-loaded foods, we will get a burst of energy that will last only a short while, and then leave us feeling more exhausted than before we ate.

If you fill your body with healthy foods such as protein, complex carbs, and healthy fats, then your body is fueled for a longer period of time, because it takes longer for our bodies to digest the healthier foods, and fuel our energy tanks for longer periods of time.

3. Greater focus

Healthy foods give us energy that helps us maintain focus, and when we eat healthy foods, we will fill our bodies and minds with greater concentration. When we consume no food, or just sugary foods, we have low energy, and reduced brain power.

4. Builds immunity

As a busy student, athlete, or just for everyday activities, it is frustrating when you have to take a day or two to nurse a cold or flu. When you eat foods that are high in vitamins and nutrients, the likelihood of you having to spend a day in bed is less likely, and even if you do get sick, you should recover from your illness much quicker than if you didn't feed your immune system with healthy options.

5. Creates good eating habits

When you settle into positive eating habits at a young age, you will be more likely to continue them as an adult. It may seem fun to eat junk food whenever you want, but that will come back to haunt you, as you become nutrient and vitamin deficient. It's fine to indulge once in a while, but maintaining clean eating will help you make better decisions, stay focused, and grow into a healthy adult.

How Diet Affects Your Mental State

Diet has a great effect on a developing mind because it gives you the sustenance for learning, and allows you to better retain information. A healthy diet also helps give you the energy to complete tasks, maintain a clear mind, and make good decisions.

Food for a Focused Mind

The foods you eat can have a huge impact on your mental well-being and your ability to make good decisions. Food has the ability to help us feel more focused and even contributes to feelings of happiness, providing we make the right choices.

Below are some foods that can help you feel more alert by providing vitamins and minerals that have proven to improve your mood, reduce stress, and help with your decision-making, by sharpening your cognitive abilities.

- **Berries** are rich in antioxidants, good at relieving stress, and can help increase your capacity to learn
- **Nuts** are not only delicious but they are full of vitamins and rich in monounsaturated and polyunsaturated fats to help with memory retention, a more alert brain, and increased oxygen levels in your bloodstream
- **Avocados** have lutein, which helps us to better understand what we are learning, and help us make better decisions
- **Eggs** are a healthy food that have many nutritional benefits, including helping your memory to retain information, and allowing your brain to function better
- **Whole grains** will help create more oxygen in the brain, which helps with memory retention,

but they will also help keep you full for a long period of time, if you have a busy school day or extra-curricular activities to go to after school

- **Greek yogurt** has minerals and vitamins that help reduce stress, and help you concentrate better

If you are old enough to take an interest in your health, chances are you are able to cook up a thing or two for yourself as well. Below are some easy-to-make recipes that will help you give yourself a good start to the day, a substantial lunch, a quick and healthy dinner, and even a tasty snack:

Ants on a log

You may have already enjoyed this simple snack. It's a great option for a quick pick-me-up that anyone can make. There really is no reason to measure or portion things out exactly, but the following recipe makes 10 servings.

Ingredients:

- 5 celery stalks
- ½ cup peanut butter (Nutella or another nut butter also works)
- ¼ cup raisins

Directions:

1. cut celery in half
2. spread peanut butter in grooves of celery
3. sprinkle with raisins

Fruit granola parfait

For a burst of energy in the morning, try this simple parfait that is quick and easy to make. Use your favorite flavor of yogurt, fruit, and granola, layered just the way you like.

Ingredients:

- ¾ cup strawberries, sliced
- ½ cup bananas, sliced
- ¾ cup blueberries
- 1 container yogurt (small/6 ounce)
- ⅓ cup granola

Directions:

1. Layer the ingredients, starting with the granola on the bottom, then fruit, then yogurt.
2. Sprinkle with 1 tbsp wheat germ, or chia seeds if you have them.

Peach Smoothie

This smoothie makes a delicious start to your day or an after-school snack. It's easy to make, with just a few ingredients.

Ingredients:

- ½ cup peach nectar
- ½ cup peaches (fresh sliced or frozen)
- ¼ cup vanilla yogurt
- 2 ice cubes

Directions:

1. Combine all ingredients in a blender, and mix until combined.

Easy bento box

There is unlimited potential to what you can include in a bento box to take to school for your lunch, and it's easy to make, so you will have no issue packing it yourself the night before school, or the morning of.

Put any of the following foods in combinations that will offer you protein, fruit, vegetables, and whole grains:

- boiled eggs (peeled)
- deli meats
- chicken
- ham
- salami
- pepperoni
- tofu
- nuts
- cheese
- cucumber
- carrots
- cherry tomatoes
- celery
- peppers
- snap peas
- grapes
- apples
- oranges
- mango

- raisins
- berries

There are several different combinations of foods you can put into these bento boxes. Make sure that all food groups are represented for a balanced meal.

Calories required

Each person will require a different amount of calories to be able to maintain a healthy weight and activity level. Caloric intake needs vary based on your age, weight, height, activity level, as well as whether or not you have stopped growing, since you will need more calories if you are still developing.

Since your body is growing and developing rapidly, it is not recommended that you try to lose weight by cutting down your caloric intake too much. Rather than deprive your body of much needed nutrients, try cutting out the foods that typically won't provide much nutrients, but will produce excessive sugar and fat reserves, such as simple carbs, sugary drinks, and processed foods.

For your health, it is essential that you do not resort to extreme measures to lose weight. Remember that your body needs a certain amount of excess fat in order to grow, and to provide your body and mind with necessary nutrients. Falling into dangerous habits such as taking diet pills or laxatives can lead to additional health problems either immediately, or in the future, such as cancer, heart disease, or other serious issues.

Don't skip meals

As a personal trainer with a wide knowledge of health and nutritional needs, I can assure you that skipping a meal will only make things more difficult for you in the long run. If you cut meals and starve your body of the calories it requires to run smoothly, you may see a drop in your weight, but this will be temporary, and may actually result in greater weight gain later on. Some ways to ensure you have a nutritional and filling meal are:

- don't skip breakfast, because this is the meal that will help jumpstart your day and give you the energy you need to get up and go
- pre-pack your lunch and fill it with healthy foods that are rich in fiber, protein, and vitamins
- help prepare the meal, and you will be able to enjoy it even more by adding your favorite flavors to it

Sleep is key

Getting enough sleep is essential for recuperating cognitive function and repairing your body, as well as allowing your food to digest, and for your body to burn through the calories that you have consumed.

Gradual is best

If you are changing your eating habits considerably, then doing it one step at a time is key. In my other books, and with my clients, I suggest making small changes to a person's daily routine, and to their eating habits, so that there is not a feeling of complete loss or being overwhelmed with the changes.

Set realistic goals

Set clear and achievable goals that you will be able to follow through on. Making small commitments to do better in any aspect of life will go well, if you have a clear path to how you will go about achieving your goals.

If you want to eat healthier but love junk food, then make a point of eating healthy all week, and saving the sugary snacks for the weekend, when you may be watching a movie, or hanging out with friends. Knowing that there is a reward down the road will help you to stay on track.

Chapter 4: The Emotional Side of Exercise

Exercise is essential for a well balanced and healthy state of mind. It is a scientifically proven fact that physical activity can also help make you happier. You may have felt a rush of excitement or energy, even euphoria after a run, hike, or playing with your sports team, but not really understood why you were having such a positive reaction. So exactly what are the emotional boosts that exercise promotes?

1. Endorphins

Exercising is proven to release endorphins, which can help relieve pain, boost mood, and significantly reduce stress. Endorphins are created in your pituitary gland and act as neurotransmitters that block out pain, and increase the feeling of happiness and pleasure. Exercise greatly increases the production of endorphins, so it is natural that working out will help you gain a sense of fulfillment and joy.

2. Dopamine

Dopamine is a neurotransmitter that helps regulate sleep cycles, heart rate, and helps to increase your ability to recall learned information, improves your mood, helps increase your attention span, and helps process pain.

3. Oxygen

As we exercise, our heart beats quicker and oxygen is pumped through our bloodstream and to our brains. When our brains are provided with ample oxygen, we are able to make better decisions, have more control over our impulses, and have a more open mind about our thinking.

Exercise also affects the cerebrum, which is where our motor functionality, intellect, and sensory impulses lie (our nerve connectivity). In the long-term, this means that cognitive functions, and the ability to maintain mobility and decision-making skills, will likely be more intact as you age.

4. Neuroplasticity

Exercise has been linked to improving neuroplasticity, which is the brain's ability to continue learning new and varied skills, such as a new language. The neural network will continue to adapt and change to learn new information by the reworking of these signaling stimuli.

All of the above benefits of exercise help your brain stay active, alert, and happy, which will in turn relieve you of feeling anxious, and can play a significant role in decreasing or preventing depression, or irrational feelings.

How Exercise Helps Your Mental State

Today's youth are under more pressure than any generation before them. There are increasing expectations for youths that they need to do it all, in order to be successful. In addition to studying and getting good grades, you are expected to anticipate your future by grade 10 in order to collect the necessary academic qualifications that prospective universities and colleges require, and that doesn't begin to touch on it.

Participating in a sport in and outside of school, going on bike rides, hikes, swimming, or using a local gym are all great ways of helping to alleviate stresses that can come with the everyday life of an adolescent. Exercise may not be able to decide your future or answer all your questions, but it will help put you in a positive state of mind, so that these expectations don't become all consuming.

Here are some examples of how exercise can help promote a healthy mental state:

1. Reduces stress

There is little doubt that the adolescent youth of today need to actively unwind to gain perspective on their hectic lives. Going for a walk, jog, bike ride, or participating in an activity that increases your heart rate and creates oxygen intake, will help clear your mind of toxic build-up, as far as negative thoughts. The release of endorphins will help deter your thoughts from any perpetual negativity you may be feeling and help sway them into a more positive way of thinking.

2. Decreased anxiety/depression

As mentioned above, exercise will help with the production and release of endorphins which are credited with making you feel happier and more positive. When you feel happy, things seem less critical and all-consuming, which will help you to see a way out of possibly devastating situations that you wouldn't have been able to before.

Anxiety brings on a host of mental discrepancies, such as depression, which make it seem impossible to overcome even the simplest of situations. By increasing endorphins, you are helping to promote a less stressful and more positive state of mind, and in turn, make more positive and productive decisions.

3. Increase memory

There is some research that links the physical activity of children to their brain development. A developing brain will retain and process information much more quickly than someone in their later years. Exercise will help you to remember what you have learned in school, may help you do better on tests, and will help protect you from possible cognitive degeneration in your older years.

4. Self-confidence

Exercise is a great way to increase serotonin levels and leave us feeling rejuvenated and fabulous. As a personal trainer, I know that my clients would begin their fitness journey feeling overwhelmed and hopeless, but after even one good workout, they felt motivated to come back. Exercise leaves you feeling great, and improves how you feel about yourself, inside and out.

Participating in group hikes, bike rides, or kayaking are only a few ways to get out and have fun connecting with others and perhaps making new friends, all while giving yourself a dose of serotonin.

5. Become more productive/creative

After a workout, I always find it easier to write about things that inspire me. Additionally, exercise helps boost your energy level so that you are more inclined to do your homework or organize your room.

6. Curbs addiction

There are many vices that are targeted towards youths today, such as vaping, alcohol, and smoking. If you are tempted to try these addictive substances, or if you have already fallen into addiction, exercise can be a good way to help you rely on a healthier addiction.

If you feel like vaping, drinking, or putting something else detrimental into your body, get outdoors, and experience the fresh air and take in nature. Look around at all the beauty that is around you, and hopefully you will feel inspired to make the healthier choice.

Get Active

The key in making good choices for yourself is to be surrounded by others who have a positive and constructive mindset. Engage with others who have the same interests as you, and who have clear goals set for their own future.

When you are in a friend group that makes bad choices such as drugs, vandalism, or reckless behavior, it may feel like you are stuck in that group, unable to make better choices without losing your whole world, but there is a way out. While the choices may be difficult, you need to walk away from negativity, and become a part of a more positive group. We tend to feel that where we are and those we know are the only way, but once you settle into a more content group, your outlook will improve.

There are several activities where you can meet new people with common interests and do the things that you love, all while promoting a healthy lifestyle.

Community involvement

A community is made up of the people that live in it, including you. Each person within a community has a role to play, and actively becoming a part of yours will allow you to grow and contribute in ways that you may not realize. Some of the benefits to being involved in your neighborhood include:

- better chance of academic success
- less chance of making poor decisions
- feelings of self-worth and a smaller likelihood of falling into a depression
- lending to more success as an adult
- providing more guidance from others in times of trouble
- there is a sense of pride and knowing you did well
- connecting with other teens who are like-minded and want to make a difference

There are unlimited pros to becoming an active member or your community but getting involved may not be apparent. Some ways you can become active and begin to make positive connections include:

- offering to tutor younger kids in subjects that you are good at
- music lessons are a great way to connect with others in your neighborhood, and you get to do what you love
- volunteer to clean a street in your neighborhood, and show your pride in where you live
- offer to read at your local library during story time for younger kids

- help an elderly person, or someone with limited abilities in your neighborhood to do chores or errands

Opening yourself up to your community, and those in it, will give you a sense of belonging and pride. Being a part of a group means that you always have people to support you, and this can make a huge difference in a youth's life.

Youth programs

Youth programs are offered in most towns and cities across the country. These programs offer opportunities to develop and grow your social skills, access a deeper connection to yourself, meet other youth, and offer programs that build leadership skills.

Your local community center should have programs available that suit a variety of interests, including kayaking, mountain biking, camping, volunteering, sports, and even dances. These opportunities will allow you to meet other tweens and teens in your area and make connections that are based on common interests.

Church groups

If you belong to a church, then you may already be aware of some of the programs that they offer to connect youth with their communities. Churches are a great place to connect with other youths, and to make plans to help out others in your city or town, volunteer to help the homeless, and may even lend to larger opportunities, such as building homes in third world countries.

Chapter 5: Your Emotional, Mental, and Physical Health

We've already touched on the importance of emotional and mental wellbeing in tweens and teens, and how important it is that you learn to nurture yourself and maintain the delicate balance between happiness and feeling overwhelmed.

When you are between the ages of 10 and 19 years old, you are entering into an exciting and formative time. Physical changes are happening to your body, seemingly overnight in some cases, and there are changes in elementary to middle school or high school, with social groups changing, and you are learning to be socially aware of those around you, and of your own actions. This time can be difficult, so it is essential that you have taken accountability for your own health, which is a great first step.

Your emotional, physical, and mental health are all connected, and so caring for all of these should be a top priority. It may seem redundant to mention emotional and mental health separately, but they are very different. Mental health is about how we take in and process the situations and events that happen to us, while emotional health is more about how we feel as a result of the information.

Emotional health

Tweens and teens go through many ups and downs as they get older, and while many of these emotional crevasses can be attributed to hormones, many more can be correlated to the fact that your life is changing more rapidly than at any other time in your life, such as:

- socializing and peer pressure
- becoming more engaged in sports and extracurricular activities
- getting part-time employment
- deciding on your college or university path
- becoming more independent and possibly clashing with authority figures

There are so many changes in your life that affect your happiness and perspective, that it can be exceedingly overwhelming. If you have decided to part ways with a friend who is going down the wrong path, this can cause feelings of guilt and grief for the loss of that friend. This is also the age that many adolescents realize that their parents or other family members whom they once saw as flawless, or a role model, may not be as perfect as they once seemed.

This is a good time to remember that while you can feel helpless or out of control, you are never alone. Become involved in a community project, join a team, or volunteer, to help you get a sense of belonging. Your feelings are valid, and your emotions are not unlike what many other adolescents are going through.

Remember to reach out if you are feeling out of control, as there are many people you can confide in, such as:

- parents
- siblings
- other family members
- school counselors
- teachers
- pastors
- doctors
- friends
- support hotlines

When things are bearing down on you, take a minute to consider alleviating some of the load. You may want to rethink your part-time job, choose your favorite extracurricular activity rather than two or three, or join a study group if you are not succeeding on your own.

Mental health

Mental health explains an umbrella of other components that are added together to make up the composition of mental health. Emotions, how we fit into society, and psychological impact is all a part of mental health, and affects how we handle stress, the decisions we make, and how we interact with and relate to others.

Throughout our entire lives, and especially in the adolescent years, mental health will change and affect us and our relationships with those we come in contact with. There are many contributing factors that fall into the umbrella of mental health issues or wellness, such as:

- brain chemistry and biological contributions
- genetics and family history of mental illness
- any abuse or trauma suffered by the individual

Often, those suffering from mental health issues won't know that anything is wrong until the symptoms become severe, and it is affecting how they deal with daily life and the most basic functions. Some signs that you are suffering from wavering health include:

- increase or decrease in sleep
- struggling to get through the day
- no interest in activities that you once loved
- becoming confrontational with friends and family
- dwelling on the past
- having the sensation of numbness
- feeling that nothing matters
- reckless behavior like drinking, smoking, or using drugs
- unexplained feelings of anxiety, sadness, anger, or irritability
- self-harm

These signs and symptoms may seem overwhelming, but if you know what you are up against, it makes it easier for you to help alleviate the situation. There are some things you can do to help your mental health:

- maintain a positive attitude
- connect with family and friends in a positive way

- get a hobby
- exercise regularly
- get 8-10 hours of sleep a night

If you are unable to find some peace in any of the above, it may be time to see a professional, and ask them to show you some coping strategies.

Physical health

Physical health is important to how well your body operates, but it also affects your mental and emotional health, as I have mentioned. Exercise not only helps you feel and look good, but it can help protect your bones from fracture, prevent osteoporosis, and can help prevent certain illnesses, including cancers.

It is recommended that every adolescent participates in physical activity for at least one hour per day, including walking, biking, participating in sports, or something else that gets you moving. For optimal benefits, it is suggested that more vigorous exercises are engaged in for at least three days a week, for the following results:

- increase heart rate, and increase air in and out of the lungs
- build stronger muscles

- increase bone strength by skipping rope, climbing on a playground, or a sport-like volleyball

You can add up shorter periods of exercise to comprise the hour each day. For example, if it takes you a half hour to walk to school and a half hour home, then that equals one hour of exercise.

Why Emotions Affect Teens So Deeply

Have you ever been called an emotional person, or had someone tell you that you are overly dramatic? The truth is that teens do tend to feel emotions more deeply, and there is a good reason for that, which begins with the limbic system.

The limbic system is responsible for our emotions; including our drive to do well, our motivation, and our acknowledgement of reward; while our frontal lobe is responsible for our impulses, social skills, decision making abilities, and our reasoning. These two systems will become more in tune with each other as you age and your brain develops.

As a child enters the teenage years, the limbic system is still developing, and the amygdala is responsible for rational thinking, but, in simple terms, it likes to send rumors through the adolescent brain, and have them feel emotions that are based on things that a more developed mind wouldn't consider an issue. This part of the brain likes to make a teenager misinterpret words and expressions for what they are not intended to be. For example, your parents might ask if you've completed your homework, but what you might hear is that you are lazy.

The prefrontal cortex is the reasoning voice that steps in at around age twenty and reassures us that there is something more reasonable going on and thoughts are not controlled through impulsive insecurity.

The teenage years are difficult enough already with your body, school, friends, responsibilities, and so much more, all changing at once. But it is the underdeveloped part of the brain that makes these things feel a lot bigger than they are.

It's important to understand that your feelings need to be validated, and you are not just being emotional because you are a teenager. Your brain is literally having you believe vicious rumors and gossip that no one has said and exaggerating the hardships that you do have. Before you react in a big way to a situation, try to give yourself a minute to breathe, and consider what you can say calmly, rather than in a harsh and abrupt way. Taking a minute to determine the extent of the situation could save you a great deal more trouble down the road.

The Power of Emotional Strength

No one should feel that they are not able to express how they feel at any time. When things become too much, there are some ways that you can help yourself regain control over your emotions without allowing them to control you.

1. Acknowledge what emotion you are feeling

Getting through any emotion is going to be easier when you know what emotion you are dealing with, so label it. Are you anxious, sad, angry, frustrated? Sometimes we misinterpret one emotion for another; for example, you may think you are angry at someone for calling you out on poor behavior, but what you are really feeling is shame or embarrassment. You don't have to admit anything to anyone but yourself, so really think about what you are feeling, and why you may be so hesitant of letting go of this emotion.

Don't be angry without your emotions because they are a part of you. Giving your feelings a name will allow you to address them better and work things out in your own way, without feeling out of control.

2. Manage your thinking

We tend to interpret news or a simple phrase based on our current mood. If you had studied for a test for weeks, and felt good about how you performed on it, you might feel really good about your teacher asking you to stay after class to talk. While, on the other hand, if you felt that you didn't study enough, the same request may leave you feeling dread, but for all you know, your teacher only wants to see if you can help them grade papers.

"I need to talk to you" can be scary words, or hopeful ones. These words might even make you feel indifferent; it all depends on your mood at the time. If you have read these words in a text after you just had a fight with your friend, then you may think more bad news is on the horizon. While if you are happy, this may seem like another wonderful bit of news.

Don't let your mood interpret the words or actions of others, and don't assume anything until you know everything for sure. Considering various scenarios is only going to serve to make you more anxious.

3. Emotional regulation

By maintaining a positive outlook on things, you are less likely to have feelings of instability. Allowing your emotions to drive your actions will lead to worries and anxieties that are not necessary. Consider the positive side of life always, and let that be your way of thinking, until you know for certain.

There will always be times when you feel underwhelmed and sad, but why put yourself through unnecessary trials and tribulation? There will be plenty of times that you will need to worry, so don't waste it on time that can be spent on positive thinking.

4. Do something to boost serotonin

When you feel discouraged with yourself or those around you, it's easy to dwell in that feeling, rather than trying to get out of it. When people are in a bad mood, they tend to complain about everything, including those around them, the weather, their job, and anything else they see around them or online. Alternatively, if someone feels happy, they see more joy and positivity in the world, as well as in the actions of others.

If you are feeling a little down, or like the world is ugly, participate in something that will help boost your mood, so that you may soon begin to see things through rose-colored glasses once again.

Chapter 6: Societal Pressures are Real

I've touched on some of the societal pressures that youths face today, but they far exceed what many consider. Adults like to say that they are swamped with work, upkeeping the home, carpooling kids, cleaning, and other valid duties that need to be completed every day, but the pressures that are put on teenagers are not often met with the same compassion, or even with any sense of acknowledgement.

Even with the outstanding number of responsibilities that teenagers face every day, you are not often taken seriously enough. The pressures of school, jobs, friends, sports; they are all taken with a grain of salt, and not nearly the same sympathy as their older family members might receive in their daily plights.

Societal pressure is ever present in a teenager's life, and it is enough to break even the strongest person.

1. Body issues

The changes that occur in the body of a teenager are enormous. You are no longer a child, and your body is changing in ways that you don't understand. To make matters worse, every magazine is graced with a beautiful cover model with flawless skin and a huge smile.

It is hard to accept your own blemishes, imperfections, and mood swings when you are being surrounded by beautiful, happy, carefree people on television, in magazines, characters in books, and on social media. Even those with weight issues online seem to be okay with it, because they are the quirky friends that everyone loves, and meanwhile you feel awkward in your own skin, and can't figure out how to fit in.

The pressure to feel secure and happy all the time is immense as a teenager, and if you don't feel like you belong, then how can you possibly find a place in this world? The most dangerous thing for teenagers' self-esteem is what social media and Hollywood hammer into them.

Even without the fantasy world of photoshop and media lies, a teenager is changing from a caterpillar into a butterfly, and the process is magical, but not every part is lovely. Be proud of your changing body and facial features, and even the cracking in your voice, and know that it's not always going to be this way. Surround yourself with people who see you for who you are and support you through your more difficult times.

2. Identity

Body issues are not the only concerns that teenagers deal with when trying to feel like they belong. As a tween or a teenager, you are finding out how your body will change in how tall you will be, how your hair color may change, how your teeth grow in, and many more details that are unique to you, and that you cannot easily change. In addition to puberty, you might be discovering who you are as a person, emotionally, mentally, and sexually.

It is common in the teenage years to discover yourself changing in a way that your friends are not. During this time, you may realize that you are angrier than others and cannot control it, or maybe you are not interested in the sex that many believe you should be pursuing. Learning that your sexuality deviates from what many others might consider normal or discovering that your mind isn't wired the way that most other teens' minds are, can be traumatic.

The teenage years are formative for your identity in all ways, and you may find that you need someone to talk to about your feelings.

3. Time management

As you age, the pressure to become more involved in school, sports, and extracurricular activities increases. With homework, socializing, and other time commitments, it's difficult to know when to find time for yourself.

You are at an age when people want you to make your own decisions, be more responsible, and take accountability for your actions, and it can be a stressful time that can lead to feelings of inadequacy, depression, and even acting out.

4. Social pressures

Parents and peers can have exceedingly high expectations for you. Your parents might feel that they weren't given the opportunities that you have had, or that they didn't live up to their potential, so it all falls on you to make good on their achievements.

Socially, your friends may be leaning toward drugs, alcohol, or other disruptive behaviors, and trying to get you to participate as well. Oftentimes, teens feel they are obligated to partake in reckless behavior, so that they keep their friends, which causes greater pressure.

5. Poor physical and mental health

Your mental and physical health is interchangeable, meaning that if you are struggling with one, you will lack in the other. Some things that can lead to further detriment of health, both mentally and physically, include:

- Sleep is important, as mentioned previously, and if a teenager is not getting at least eight hours of sleep a night, they will go through their day on an energy deficit
- Nutrition is important because if you are not supplying your body with ample nutrients and vitamins, then you will be running on a deficit in that department as well, and not have enough energy to get through the day without feeling completely haggard
- Anxiety and depression are associated with stress, hormone changes, and expectations put

upon us, which can also show in a lack of patience toward others, or anger toward them

6. Bullying

Remarkably, one in three teens in North America have been bullied in one form or another. Bullying can happen indirectly or directly, by either purposefully telling, being verbally or physically abusive to someone, or through gossip-spreading lies.

The effects of someone attacking you on social media can be devastating and should be taken very seriously.

7. Drugs

Drugs are more prevalent today than ever before, and dealers are targeting teenagers with their products by making them seem more appealing in the form of candies. The pressure from peers can be exhausting when you are young because you want to fit in, but may be struggling with the ethical dilemma, as well as what it could potentially do to your health.

How to Deal with Others' Expectations

Unrealistic expectations are often projected on a teenager when someone is feeling inadequate about their own accomplishments. Whether it's your parents, grandparents, teachers, or other influential persons in your life, the high expectations that are shuffled onto a child are often because they were unable to achieve what they wanted to in their own youth, or even in their life at this time.

When you are being urged to do something that you are not enjoying or that you never had interest in, chances are someone forced or strongly suggested you be a part of it. They may be the ones pushing you to join the team you want nothing to do with or work the job you never wanted. There needs to come a time when you follow your own interests, rather than what someone else wants for you.

There is a certain level of reasonable expectations that a parent may want to see from their children, but when it comes to pushing a child beyond their limits, that expectation may become unrealistic.

Not everyone is an academic genius, so if you are trying your best by studying for exams, completing your homework assignments, and participating in class, but still not getting grades that your parents are proud of, they are setting you up with unrealistic expectations. An athlete who practices hours each day and still doesn't lure college prospects cannot be told they are not striving to be their best selves.

The unrealistic goals that others put on you, whether academic, job-oriented, or in sports, are not on you to live up to. Do the best you can and voice your wishes if you feel that someone is trying to press their own agenda on you.

You may want to make your parents proud by playing a sport they love or majoring in a subject that they pursued, but if it doesn't make you happy, and if it isn't your path, let them know the interests that you do have. For you to be happy and follow your own path toward goals you want to attain, you need to explore your options, make your own mistakes, and accept that you may have to veer away from the way you and others once expected of you.

The Power of Positivity

Positive thinking is key when it comes to living a happy life. Cultivating positivity in all that you do will help you to make better choices and treat yourself better. A positive lifestyle begins by making the choice to do better and live happier every day. Rarely is anyone born to naturally think the best in everyone, to believe in themselves unconditionally, and to believe that everything is going to always be okay. You need to make the choice each morning to do whatever you can to boost your serotonin levels by exercising, appreciating people for their efforts, giving praise, and being thankful.

There are some ways that you can promote positivity in your daily life that are likely to be habitual as you move forward in your life, and become a habit, rather than something you need to think about. Some of the habits and choices of positive people include:

1. Surrounding yourself with positive people

Just as a negative person can succeed in bringing you into a darker mind set, a positive person can help to influence you to be a better role model in your own life, as well as in the lives of others. Focus on spending your time with people who build others up, rather than find faults in them.

You may not know exactly where to begin in your journey to finding a positive group of friends, especially if you have just removed yourself from people prone to negative thinking. Someone who is trying to promote positivity may be involved in volunteering, so looking into a group where you can help out is a good place to start.

People who are more successful tend to have a positive mindset. Rarely do people with a negative attitude do well in a professional or group setting, because they find it difficult to get along with others, and their outlook and goals are not as strong.

2. Choose your words carefully

The words you use can help determine the path of success you go down, as well as help you when pursuing your goals. If you want to be successful in anything, you need to use powerful words that express your determination and the belief you have in yourself. If you continually tell yourself that you aren't doing well in a subject, or that you will not play well in the game, that will work its way into your subconscious and beat down your ability to be successful.

Pay attention to the words you use and stop yourself whenever you notice that you are speaking down on yourself or using words that do not promote prosperity or success. Instead of using words such as *can't*, *unable*, *fail*, or any other negative way to describe yourself or something you do, choose a positive word to put in its place. For example, rather than saying, *I am so bad at science*, try saying, *I will try my best in science*. The spin on your words may have a surprising result on a more positive outcome.

You may have heard of daily affirmations, and I can tell you from experience, they do work. Set yourself up each day with an affirmation of hope and success by using phrases such as:

- I am a kind and positive person who attracts positive people
- I am proud of my accomplishments and of the accomplishments of my friends

- My positive outlook will help guide me toward more positive people

If you need to prepare yourself for a job interview or get in a positive mindset for a game or a test, recite to yourself powerful phrases that reassure you that you are enough, you have a lot to offer, and that you will do your best.

Those who believe they will succeed and will do their best every day to surround them with positive peers and role models, are more likely to succeed in relationships, careers, and in taking care of their overall wellness.

Chapter 7: When You Can't Do It All

Feeling like you have too much on your plate and that you can't keep up is frustrating, but it is also completely normal. Life is busy, and the more you want to make of it, the more difficult it is to find the time to see it all through.

When you are feeling overwhelmed, it is a good time to remember your positive affirmations, and tell yourself that you can do it, even when the lack of time is making you feel like you can't do it all. From experience in my own life, as well as with coaching my clients through their own difficulties, I've found the following tips help make everything seem a bit more achievable:

1. Be persistent

Persistence in life is key to success. It is near impossible to achieve any goal without making the effort to persist despite any obstacles. Becoming a part of the debate club or basketball team might be mandatory in elementary gym class, but if you want to really hone in on your skills, you have to practice and go through trial and errors.

If you expect that everything will come easily and are the type to give up when things become more difficult, then you are not likely to succeed. When things become a challenge, you need to put in more effort by practicing for longer hours, doing more research, studying every day; whatever you are trying to achieve is worth the extra time.

It may be difficult to do it all, but it's not impossible as long as you have set your achievable goals and have not taken on more activities and responsibilities than a 24 hour day allows. Your daily affirmation shouldn't be *I can't do it all,* but rather, *I can do this.*

2. Address your opponent

In this scenario, your opponents are time and achievement, and you may feel that you don't have enough time to tackle the achievements you set out to conquer. The first thing you need to do when you feel that you are unable to do it all is to address why you feel that way; only then can you figure out how to overcome it.

Address the issues that are preventing you from achieving your goals, and then tackle them one by one. For example, if you want to try to get to college on a basketball scholarship, but also need to work part-time to earn money for college, you are likely going to run into the challenge of finding time for both. These are real challenges that some teens face, and for it all to work out, there needs to be a well-formulated solution.

Addressing the issues that you face, whether time related, or that you just feel you lack certain skills, will give you an idea of how to get around those challenges. Where there is a will, there is a determined youth that is going to find a way to get it done, but you need to address the issues in order to work beyond them.

3. One step at a time

One of the first things we learn in life is how to walk, and that is done by literally taking one step at a time. When we look toward our goals or at what needs to be done through the day, week, or month, it's easy to become overwhelmed when looking at everything together. The best way to look at a group of seemingly impossible tasks is to take a page from your younger self, and to break them down, and take it step by step.

When we look at even the most monumental obstacles and tasks individually, rather than all at once, we can see these challenges as stepping stones that we need to take one at a time to help get us to our goal.

Look at it as running four laps at the track; thinking about running 1600 meters can exhaust you before you've set a foot over the starting line, but if you focus on getting to the first 100 meter line, then the second, then third, and fourth, until you complete your first lap, it becomes more manageable.

You may wake up with a feeling of failure before the day begins because you can't imagine how you will get through your day. Rather than looking toward the night when it's all done, focus on the first thing you need to do; what is the immediate task at hand? Worry about the next step after the first is complete, or you will become tangled in a web of missteps and find it hard to gain traction. You can get through your day if you pre-plan and take it one step at a time.

4. Accept change

You need to remember that not everything in life will go smoothly, nor will it always be as you imagined. Accept that sometimes there will be challenges that cannot be overcome and consider what can be done differently to help you get back on the right path.

Don't get discouraged when you need to make alterations in your plans or that things may take a little longer to achieve than you thought. Sometimes, life throws us curve balls and it's up to you to catch them or allow them to take you out. Keep going on the path you choose and understand that not everything worth getting will be easy.

Dealing with Mounting Pressures

Being aware of the pressures that you are under and how they will affect you can be beneficial in helping you develop coping strategies. You may not even realize how stressed you have become with all that you are expected to accomplish in a week with school, work, sports, peers, volunteering, or anything else you have on the go. There are some signs that you should be aware of that will help you determine if you are under mounting pressure:

1. Exhaustion

If you hit the snooze button every morning and still feel exhausted, even after getting a full night's sleep, it may be that you are literally physically exhausted. Stress sends signals through the rest of your body that it needs to work overtime to fix whatever is wrong; only, it doesn't know exactly what to fix. Your body will continue working on alleviating the stress until it is depleted, which is only possible if you figure out a way to lower the stress levels.

2. Insomnia

The real kicker is that stress can make you feel exhausted when you get sleep, but it can also prevent you from getting the rest that you so desperately need. When you are worried, your mind races through the various problems that you are dealing with and makes it difficult to get any rest, therefore leaving you feeling tired, on top of being physically depleted.

3. Chronic pain

As mentioned above, your body does not do well under stress, despite it putting every effort into dealing with it. Your body will work to fix the issue which only puts additional strain on your emotional state, as well as your physical well-being.

When your mind is stressed, your body will tense up as well, leaving your muscles strained, and your head and body aching, too. For such a miraculous system, the human body cannot appreciate that it is your mind putting it through the anguish. The best thing to do is to calm yourself and try to put at least some of your stressors out of your mind.

4. Frequent illness

Our immune systems need sleep in order to heal anything that is ailing, so when we don't get proper sleep, we have not given our bodies enough time to become well. With your body greeting diversions through worry, you are likely to have difficulty fending off even a common cold, and once you are sick, the recovery time will be increased significantly due to the depleted immune system.

5. Becoming forgetful

When you are feeling overwhelmed, it is likely that your thoughts are focused on many things that are pressing, which leaves little space in your brain to remember everything. You may find that you forget to complete or hand in assignments, forget appointments or plans with friends, or wander from one room to the next without a clue why you made the trip.

6. Dizziness

Breathing is literally the most important and natural thing we do in our lives, but many of us forget to breathe properly when we are stressed, which could lead to panic attacks and feeling dizzy. As natural as it is, we often forget to breathe properly when we are stressed, and take in short, shallow breaths that make us feel anxious.

Taking too much on can make a huge impact on your physical, mental, and emotional health, so you need to make sure that you take time for yourself and develop coping strategies to help keep you feeling calm.

Make Your Health a Priority

There is only one of you in this world, and you are very important to many people, even if it doesn't always feel that way. There are a lot of things in the life of a tween or teen that are enough to make a grown man go mad, so acknowledge that you are doing a lot, and allow yourself to prioritize *you.*

There are some simple ways that you can reduce your stress and take a break from the chaos to feel calm again:

1. Laughing

Laughter is the best medicine, for real, because it releases cortisol, dopamine, epinephrine, and endorphins, all of which make you feel happier. Laughter also helps strengthen our immune systems by enhancing T cells, which help to boost our immune systems.

2. Walking

Going for a walk and enjoying nature is one of the best things you can do for your mental health. Take in the scenery and the creatures that live in it and allow your thoughts to be overwhelmed with peaceful nature, and leave your anxious thoughts behind. Take deep breaths of the fresh air, and really think about your breaths as you inhale and exhale evenly and deeply.

3. Waking earlier

Especially if you are feeling overwhelmed with too little time in the day, getting up earlier will provide more hours in your day to get more accomplished. If you are up early enough to get some things off your to-do list, then you are going to feel less overwhelmed throughout the day.

4. Eating well

Since the food you eat fuels your body, make sure you are choosing healthy options, such as whole grains, especially in the morning, so your body can use the nutrients throughout the day and keep your energy levels up.

5. Visiting friends

When you are feeling overwhelmed, getting in touch with friends to go for a meal, watch a movie, or just talk can help take your mind off your worries and give you some quality time away from your thoughts.

Chapter 8: When You Change Your Path

As we grow, our interests change, and we may realize that what we have been chasing isn't really what we were meant to do after all. Even if you have been chasing the dream that you will go to college on a basketball scholarship, it's okay to decide that you don't want to spend the next four years of your life devoted to one thing. Changing careers is something that many adults do after a decade or two, so it makes sense that the same opportunity be made available to a teenager who is exploring their options for the first time.

A reason for a change of heart where your extracurriculars or college majors are concerned, is that you have suffered an injury that took away your athletic scholarship, or the opportunity to try. As devastating as this loss may be, you need to take into account that things change, and life doesn't always go your way, so the only option left is to focus your talents on something else.

There is no shame in reevaluating your goals. Often, we have more than one passion and it takes time and maturity to decide which we would like to pursue. It is possible that you may change your mind on a career halfway through college, but that doesn't mean that you failed, it only means that you have built a foundation of knowledge on which you will nurture a new development in your life. Time invested in yourself is never a waste, so if you have redirected your goals, embrace the decision, and move onward.

When life sets you on a path you never expected to be on, you need to be thankful that you can reset your goals and start anew. Take into consideration that not everyone gets a second, or even a first chance. There are many obstacles that could have played a part, but all you can do is take a moment to acknowledge that things didn't work out and move on.

Accepting Failure

It may not be in your playbook to accept failure, as many people are unwilling to accept that they weren't able to accomplish what they set out to do. Failure can come in many forms, from a failed relationship to a grade that wasn't as good as you expected, or not making the team that you tried out for.

Failure is a part of life, and it helps us to become better for having learned to be flexible. While you will learn to deal with rejection and disappointment, there are some ways that may help you to cope with a change of plans.

It may be normal to fail, but that doesn't change the fact that it's a scary thing to deal with, especially for teenagers. What makes failure so scary for a teen may be because of:

- wanting to present a perfect life on social media platforms
- wanting to live up to a parent's expectations
- academic achievements and the pressure to get a high GPA
- getting a job to save up for a car, college, or even help at home

When there is a risk of imminent failure or when a teenager has not done as well as they should have, there are many ways with which they can react, including:

- self-inflicted injuries
- depression or anxiety becoming an issue
- withdrawal from social activities
- self-loathing
- anger toward others or feelings of irritability

Today, many people are calling for the normalization of mental illness, asking for help, and self-love, so why don't we also normalize failure? With the likelihood of failure so high in one's lifetime, it stands to reason that we should be more accepting of it, and embrace it as a learning experience, rather than feeling shame. Failure is mislabeled, as far as I'm concerned, since the only failure that someone truly faces is not trying in the first place.

What We Can Learn from Our Darkest Times

In difficult times, it is important to give yourself credit for every step you took to get through them. It takes great strength to go through something emotionally, mentally, or physically draining, and come out the other side ready to try again. There are some important take-aways that you should consider when you are going through a dark time or have come through a dark time.

1. You are strong

Give yourself credit for facing a new day. With the intense pressure that youths are under today, sometimes it's all you can do to get out of bed and start anew. Feeling depleted and sad or angry does not mean you are weak. Getting up and challenging a new day shows strength and determination.

2. Everyone struggles

You are not alone in your struggles, even if they feel excessive. There is always an opportunity to reach out for help, as long as you acknowledge that you are not flawed. We often want to hide our struggles because mental illness and trauma is often talked about in hushed voices, and followed by, "but don't say anything." Why not tell people you are having a hard time? Mental illness affects one in five youth, and not all of them get the help they need, because they feel ashamed. Mental illness isn't a bad word, and it does not mean that you are damaged; it just means that you need help to get to a better place.

3. All storms pass

Your life may seem tumultuous right now, but I can tell you from experience that it will pass. It is a challenge to see beyond the teenage years to a time when you won't struggle or feel different, but there will come that day. Hold on and know that you are worth your time and space on this earth.

Chapter 9: Asking for Help

As an adult, I can tell you that no one gets through life without asking for help. Helping others is a natural part of life, and something you likely do for others without even thinking about it. Asking for and giving help is what literally helps us build strong relationships. Sometimes asking for help can be a difficult thing to do, especially if you were raised to deal with your own problems. Our egos often stand in our way of getting the help that we need, but there are common misconceptions that you need to overcome.

1. Sign of weakness

Asking for help is actually a sign of strength, because it shows great maturity to realize you need a hand, and it takes courage to reach out to someone. Asking for help doesn't mean you cannot get by on your own, it means that you will learn better, or be more successful with some help.

2. You're not worthy

Everyone deserves to be given a hand or lent support sometimes. We all struggle and reaching out to others can help us build more of a support system.

3. Afraid to speak up

Be direct when you need help, rather than milling around and not saying what you mean, as this can be frustrating. Approach your friend, parent, or teacher with, "I need help with _____. Can you help me?"

4. Waiting for someone to ask

If you are waiting for someone to ask why you are struggling, you may not ever get help. People may care a great deal about your happiness, but if you aren't willing to open up, they may not want to pry. Rather than waiting for someone to ask you what's wrong, let them in on what's got you down so they can help.

5. Giving up

There's no doubt that it can be easier to give up on getting help than pushing onward. Not every problem is going to be solved with your first attempt. You may need to explain your situation more than once, or ask a few people, before you get the help you need. Persevere rather than give up on yourself; you're worth the effort.

Asking for help is an important step in one's personal development. Just as you might wish for someone to reach out to you, don't be afraid to offer your support to someone you think might need it. Without being nosey, you could say, "I've noticed you aren't quite yourself. I'm here if you want to talk." Lending your support could make a huge difference in someone's life.

Nothing Is Strong Without a Supportive Foundation

Relationships are built piece by piece, and the strongest ones are built on a foundation of trust and respect that has been constructed over a period of time. We need to offer all sides of ourselves if we want to have deep connections in our lives.

When we only talk about topical issues or keep things impersonal, there is no real basis for trust and respect and our relationships are likely to crumble. When we allow ourselves to be vulnerable and invite others to do the same, we become raw in order to become stronger, with the help of those we choose to have around us.

When you consider confiding in someone, it helps if you know they will keep your trust and not share your secrets. A good way to recognize if someone is going to keep your confidence is to recognize if they gossip or spread rumors about other people. If they are not kind toward others, or if they share information that they have been asked to keep, they are likely not going to keep anything you tell them private.

Supporting Others

Building a strong idea of yourself and helping to create a well-rounded perspective includes you supporting others. As mentioned, ask a friend if they could use someone to talk to, or offer to study with a friend who is struggling.

Supporting others can also include volunteer work in your community. Retirement homes, hospitals, after-school care programs, or other local affiliations are always looking for help in various capacities. Offer to dish out meals at a soup kitchen or run a day camp for younger kids during the summer.

Putting yourself in a position to help others will give you a deeper sense of accomplishment and will help build your community.

Chapter 10: Embracing Your Health

The initiative to take your health seriously is a huge step that needs to be commended. We have gone through how foods, exercise, and surrounding yourself in a positive environment will help you to maintain optimal health.

Embracing your health is not just about eating healthy, though; it is about taking care of your mental health as well. Having a strong sense of self and strengthening your mind is also about exploring different things and finding out what truly makes you happy.

For most of your life you have been introduced to people, activities, and places that adults in your life thought you would enjoy. All the experiences you have gone through have helped to mold you into the amazing person you are today, but some of them may not have been your first choice. Now that you are older, take the time to find out what really interests you, and learn to introduce your own boundaries for people, as you have been taught to respect boundaries for your whole life.

Some ways to help find your true interests and help support all aspects of your health include:

1. Exploring your surroundings

Go on adventures that you haven't already experienced. There are many ways to find local trails, water sports, youth groups, and anything else, just by entering a few words into Google.

Before you make any absolute decisions, talk with your parents or caregiver about what you would like to try. If you aren't sure what you want to explore, ask them to help you find outings based on your interests. Expanding your horizons may bring you to the conclusion that you've been focusing on the wrong sport, or school major, and maybe you were meant to do something else.

When you limit your experiences, you are limiting your potential. Open up your mind to the opportunities that may arise from really getting to know your neighborhood or your city.

2. Opening a dialogue

Be open to allowing others in your family to join you on adventures and outings, because you may find that it's a great way to connect with them, and help open up a dialogue for conversations that are difficult to have otherwise.

One of the reasons that teenagers feel they have no one to turn to is because they have never been able to say the hard things out loud. If you don't spend time with your siblings, parents, or friends, chances are your dialogue is superficial, meaning you talk about school, sports, chores, and little else. By spending quality time with people, you are opening up a greater dialogue that can open up real avenues of discussion.

Ask your parents about their youth and what they were interested in and let them in on some of the issues you face. Asking their opinion may actually be helpful. Despite growing up in a very different time, your parents were once teenagers, too. Opening up to others about a serious issue is much easier when you can say, "remember when I told you about Jenny," or "you mentioned you had lots of friends, but did you ever feel left out?"

Having a backstory to build from when discussing serious matters is easier than if you are going to someone that you barely spend time with. Learning about other's experiences and allowing them into your own will help you to build a trust and a history of stories that you may find relatable.

3. Doing what you love

Often, a teenager is so busy focusing on what will help them get into a good college that they forget to do things they actually enjoy. Many colleges are looking for people who are outgoing, willing to work hard, and have a wide variety of interests, but they are not asking you to have *their* interests.

A college or university wants to know who they will be accepting into their establishment, and that the student will work hard. You can show them that you are able to really focus on a topic and do well by pursuing what you love, not what you think they want to see.

Remember that the endgame of life is to be happy, and should not be about pleasing others, and that includes a school.

If you have a passion for music, hone in on that love, and if you want to include this on a college application in some capacity, try volunteering to teach students in your neighborhood, especially underprivileged kids that may not be able to afford lessons to pursue what they love. Seeing that you have shared your passion with others is going to look good on a college or job application, and it will help you feel fulfilled and happy as a person, which we know leads to more stable mental health and well-being.

Stand Up for Your Health

It can be difficult when you are a kid to make healthier choices because you don't buy the groceries or make the meals, but that doesn't mean that you can't get your two cents in. Ask your parents if you can help with the grocery shopping, and if you can help in preparing meals, or at least a part of the meal.

Your health is important, and so are you. Don't be afraid to ask to be a part of producing a healthier menu for your family and implementing food choices that will help benefit both you and them.

Choosing to eat healthier foods and drinks and become more physically active will go a long way. Some small changes you can make to implement successful habits include:

- staying away from sugary drinks, including most juice; drink oat milk, or another healthy, low calorie beverage (water is always best)
- taking less food that you think you will eat; when we are hungry, we tend to heap our plates and try to finish it all
- eating slowly; try placing your utensils down after each bite, so the food has time to reach your stomach. If you eat fast, you will eat too much, and then feel stuffed and likely get a stomachache
- loading up on salad and proteins rather than potatoes, rice, and pasta

If you are eating out, don't feel obligated to eat everything that is offered. Politely let your host know that you are trying to cut down on certain foods to help yourself feel healthier. It is okay not to eat everything that is offered to you, and likely, your host will understand.

You Are Worth it

It might be easier to consider how you would feel if someone told your best friend, your sibling, or your parents that they weren't good enough, or didn't deserve to be kind to themselves. You would likely step in, and say that your friend was worth self-care, or that your sibling was amazing, no matter how many times they said otherwise. Now take that same compassion and speak those words of encouragement and support that you have for others toward yourself.

When you stop judging yourself harshly and accept that you are doing your best, you may find that your self-esteem improves, and you are given a boost of confidence to try again. Studies have found that teenagers who give themselves the proper self-care that they deserve, are more likely to succeed in their job, school, and with personal relationships.

When we take the time to appreciate ourselves through self-affirmation, meditation, exercise, or just taking time to read a book, we are telling ourselves that we are worth the time. Having a clear sense of your worth will help you stand up for yourself and make positive decisions in your life.

Conclusion

Your investment in your health is commendable and encompasses your physical, emotional, and mental wellbeing. Now that we have gone through the various changes that happen in the adolescent years, and what you need to help you to not only cope, but thrive, the only thing left is to begin your journey toward a healthier life.

The choices you make as you move toward adulthood will determine a smoother path or a more challenging time. Sometimes we struggle, even with good intentions and hard work, but having the tools at hand to help us feel more grounded, healthy, and understanding, can make the difference between barely getting by, and succeeding in life.

A well-rounded individual is one who sets goals for themselves, works diligently, and takes care of their body and mind. Our physical, mental, and emotional requirements are not independent of one another, but encapsulate us in entirety. To have a healthy body and mind, we need to eat healthy foods, participate in physical activities, and find time to socialize with those who make us happy.

Balancing the chemicals in your brain with the help of exercise and balanced meals will help prevent depression and anxiety, but it is not guaranteed. If you feel you are struggling despite your best efforts, it may be time to consider speaking to a professional about your mental health.

Your Body, Your Mind, Your Business

The choice to better your mental, physical and emotional health is entirely up to you. You do not need to explain your decision for betterment to anyone. Someone struggling with their own health may be critical of your decision to become healthier. It is not up to you to convince them that you are right, and you don't need to spend the energy on explaining why you feel you are right. Your choices to strengthen your body and mind are personal and unique to you, therefore your opinion is the only one that matters.

If you are struggling to find happiness or peace in your mind despite your best efforts, there is no shame in asking for help from a counselor, or other medical professional. We all struggle with finding happiness from time to time, and may not be positive every single day, but if you are experiencing sadness, anxiety, or other negative feelings for longer than 2 weeks, it may be indicative of a mental health issue that can only be managed with professional help.

Taking Yourself Seriously When Others Don't

There is no one on this earth that is more important than anyone else, or who deserves to be treated more kindly, or taken more seriously. You are the only you that will ever be in this world, and you deserve to be treated with respect, and have your decisions acknowledged and validated.

The journey through life is filled with many obstacles, but as long as you know that you are worth the effort, you are likely to succeed. Challenge yourself to do better, and once you have done as much as you can, accept that maybe this is how things should be, and make the best of what you have.

When you stumble, remember that you were not born running, and that you had to fall and trip many times before you found solid ground. You have not gone through every obstacle or challenge in life yet, so when a new situation arises, give yourself time to figure it out, and if things don't go smoothly, pick yourself up and try again.

Channel your younger self when you feel like giving up, or you feel you don't deserve what you set out to accomplish. You began your life knowing how to breathe and cry, and little else. Challenge yourself to discover new things and to enjoy every step, just as you did as a toddler. You are amazing, and you deserve every bit of happiness and health you can muster.

Taking accountability for your health is going to help you to feel better and become more productive in the long run. It won't happen overnight, but with determination and a bit of time, you can gain control of your overall health.

References

American College of Neuropsychopharmacology.
(2017, December 6). *Lack of sleep could cause
mood disorders in teens*. ScienceDaily. Retrieved
from:
https://www.sciencedaily.com/releases/2017/12/1
71206090624.htm

American Sleep Association. (2017, February 3).
Stages of Sleep: The Sleep Cycle. American Sleep
Association. Retrieved from:
https://www.sleepassociation.org/about-
sleep/stages-of-sleep/

Centers for Disease Control and Prevention. (2021,
January 25). *Why It Matters*. CDC. Retrieved from:
https://www.cdc.gov/nutrition/about-
nutrition/why-it-
matters.html#:~:text=Good%20nutrition%20is%2
0essential%20in%20keeping%20current%20and

Cespedes Feliciano, E. M., Quante, M., Rifas-Shiman,
S. L., Redline, S., Oken, E., & Taveras, E. M. (2018,
July 1). *Objective Sleep Characteristics and
Cardiometabolic Health in Young Adolescents*.

Pediatrics, 142 (1).
https://doi.org/10.1542/peds.2017-4085

Clarke, G., & Harvey, A. G. (2012, April). *The Complex Role of Sleep in Adolescent Depression*. Child and Adolescent Psychiatric Clinics of North America, 21 (2), 385–400.
https://doi.org/10.1016/j.chc.2012.01.006

Dreher, M. L., & Davenport, A. J. (2013, May 2). *Hass Avocado Composition and Potential Health Effects*. Critical Reviews in Food Science and Nutrition, 53 (7), 738–750.
https://doi.org/10.1080/10408398.2011.556759

Jennison, S. (2020, December 11). *Emotional Health vs. Mental Health: The Real Difference*. Eddins Counseling Group. Retrieved from:
https://eddinscounseling.com/emotional-health-vs-mental-health/

Gavin, MD, M. (n.d.). *What Sleep Is and Why All Kids Need It*. KidsHealth. Retrieved February 18, 2022, from: https://www.kidshealth.org/en/kids/not-tired.html

Harvard Health Publishing. (2014, July 16). *What meditation can do for your mind, mood, and health*. Harvard Health Publishing. Retrieved

from: https://www.health.harvard.edu/staying-
healthy/what-meditation-can-do-for-your-mind-
mood-and-health-

Health.com. (2013, April 26). *The Best Diets For Your Skin*. Health.com. Retrieved from:
https://www.health.com/beauty/the-best-diets-
for-your-skin?slide=00a1c83c-79b6-443d-a699-
50d74df345ac#00a1c83c-79b6-443d-a699-
50d74df345ac

HealthLink BC. (n.d.). *Physical Activity for Children and Teens*. HealthLink BC. Retrieved February 26, 2022, from: https://www.healthlinkbc.ca/health-
topics/physical-activity-children-and-teens

Kumar, B., Robinson, R., & Till, S. (2015). *Physical activity and health in adolescence*. Clinical Medicine Journal, 15 (3), 267–272.
https://doi.org/10.7861/clinmedicine.15-3-267

McMakin, D. L., Dahl, R. E., Buysse, D. J., Cousins, J. C., Forbes, E. E., Silk, J. S., ... Franzen, P. L. (2016, June 15). *The impact of experimental sleep restriction on affective functioning in social and nonsocial contexts among adolescents*. Journal of Child Psychology and Psychiatry, 57 (9), 1027–1037. https://doi.org/10.1111/jcpp.12568

Morin, A. *3 Powerful Ways to Gain Control Over Your Emotions*. Psychology Today. (n.d.). Retrieved from https://www.psychologytoday.com/us/blog/what-mentally-strong-people-dont-do/201903/3-powerful-ways-gain-control-over-your-emotions

National Institute of Neurological Disorders and Stroke. (n.d.) *Brain Basics: Understanding Sleep*. National Institute of Neurological Disorders and Stroke. Retrieved from: https://www.ninds.nih.gov/disorders/patient-caregiver-education/understanding-sleep#:~:text=Most%20of%20your%20dreaming%20occurs%20during%20REM%20sleep%2C

The National Institute on Drug Abuse. (2021, February 16). *Nurturing My Mental & Emotional Health*. NIDA for Teens. Retrieved from: https://teens.drugabuse.gov/teachers/lessonplans/nurturing-my-mental-emotional-health

Reichelt, A. C., & Rank, M. M. (2017, December 18). *The impact of junk foods on the adolescent brain*. Birth Defects Research, 109 (20), 1649–1658. https://doi.org/10.1002/bdr2.1173

Rudy, L. (2022, February 4). *The Neurodivergent Brain: Everything You Need to Know.* VeryWellHealth. Retrieved from: https://www.verywellhealth.com/neurodivergent-5216749

Shieck, M. (2020, April 10). *14 Easy, Healthy Snacks Kids Can Make.* All recipes. Retrieved from: https://www.allrecipes.com/gallery/easy-healthy-snacks-kids-can-make-2/?utm_campaign=social-share-article&utm_content=20200212&utm_medium=social&utm_source=pinterest.com&utm_term=undefined&slide=da0618d1-c19b-4e64-976a-5af2dc6cc6c3#da0618d1-c19b-4e64-976a-5af2dc6cc6c3

Suni, E. (2022, January 31). *Teens and Sleep.* Sleep Foundation. Retrieved from: https://www.sleepfoundation.org/teens-and-sleep

Tarokh, L., Saletin, J. M., & Carskadon, M. A. (2016, November). *Sleep in adolescence: Physiology, cognition and mental health.* Neuroscience & Biobehavioral Reviews, 70, 182–188. https://doi.org/10.1016/j.neubiorev.2016.08.008

Taste of Home. (n.d.) *Ginger-Kale Smoothies*. Taste
of Home. Retrieved February 20, 2022, from:
https://www.tasteofhome.com/recipes/ginger-
kale-smoothies/

U.S. Department of Health & Human Services. (2020,
May 28). *What Is Mental Health?*.
MentalHealth.gov. Retrieved from:
https://www.mentalhealth.gov/basics/what-is-
mental-health

World Health Organization. (2021, November 17).
Adolescent mental health. World Health
Organization. Retrieved from:
https://www.who.int/news-room/fact-
sheets/detail/adolescent-mental-
health#:~:text=Physical%2C%20emotional%20an
d%20social%20changes%2C%20including%20exp
osure%20to

www.ingramcontent.com/pod-product-compliance
Lightning Source LLC
Chambersburg PA
CBHW050220270326
41914CB00003BA/494

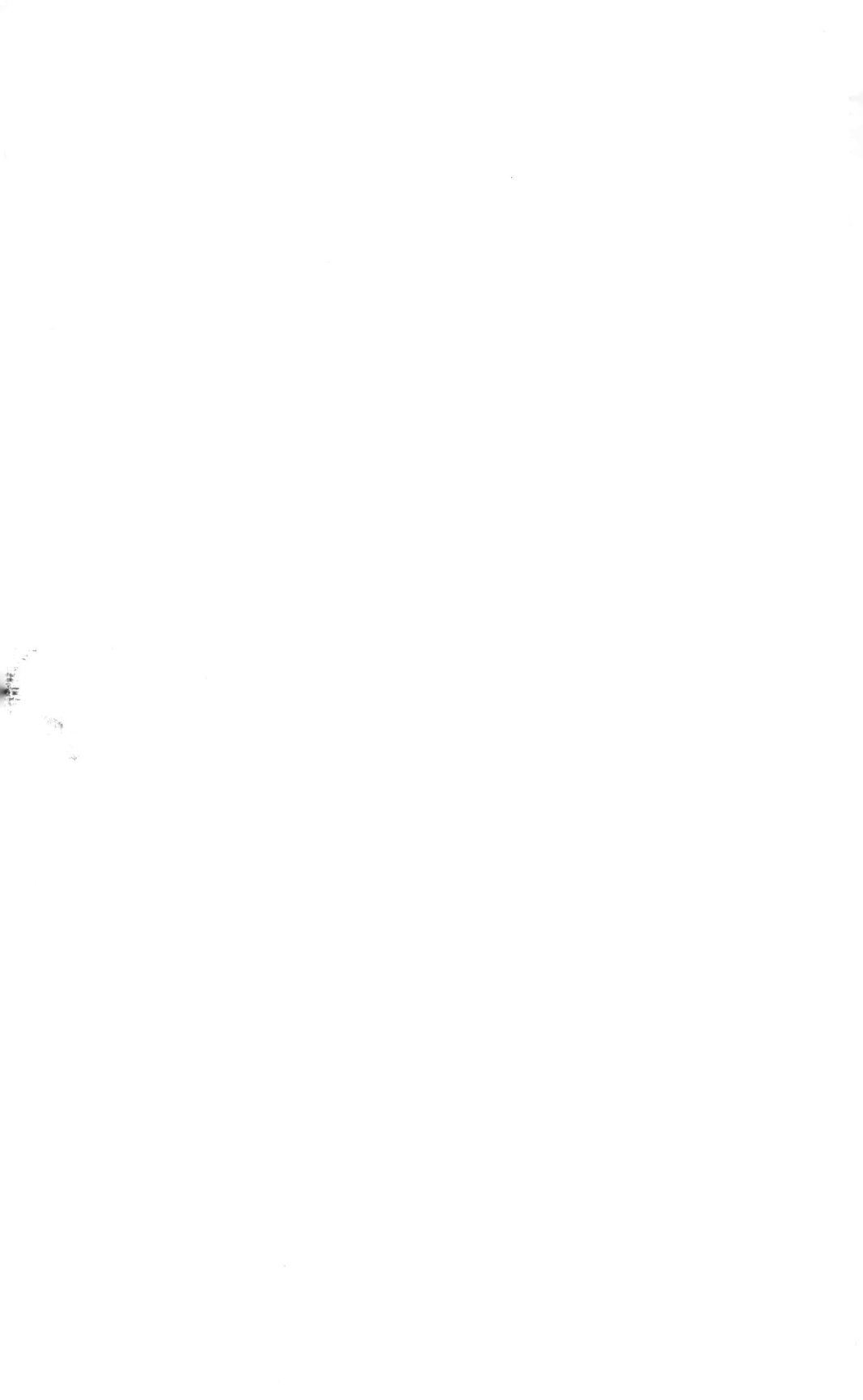